616.9

The British Medical Association
FAMILY DOCTOR GUIDE to
EPILEPSY

D0807757

The British Medical Association

FAMILY DOCTOR GUIDE *to*

EPILEPSY

DR. M. WALKER AND
PROFESSOR S. SHORVON

MEDICAL EDITOR
DR. TONY SMITH

DORLING KINDERSLEY
LONDON • NEW YORK • SYDNEY • MOSCOW
www.dk.com

IMPORTANT

This book is not designed as a substitute for personal medical advice but as a supplement to that advice for the patient who wishes to understand more about his/her condition.

Before taking any form of treatment **YOU SHOULD ALWAYS CONSULT YOUR MEDICAL PRACTITIONER.**

In particular (without limit) you should note that advances in medical science occur rapidly and some of the information contained in this book about drugs and treatment may very soon be out of date.

PLEASE NOTE

The authors regret that they cannot enter into any correspondence with readers.

A DORLING KINDERSLEY BOOK
www.dk.com

Senior Editor Mary Lindsay
Senior Designer Sarah Hall
Production Assistant Elizabeth Cherry

Managing Editor Stephanie Jackson
Managing Art Editor Nigel Duffield

Produced for Dorling Kindersley Limited by
Design Revolution, Queens Park Villa,
30 West Drive, Brighton, East Sussex BN2 2GE
Editorial Director Ian Whitelaw
Art Director Fiona Roberts
Editor Julie Whitaker
Designer Vanessa Good

Published in Great Britain in 1999 by
Dorling Kindersley Limited,
9 Henrietta Street, London WC2E 8PS

2 4 6 8 10 9 7 5 3 1

A CIP catalogue record for this book is available from the British Library

ISBN 07513 0682 7

Reproduced by Colourscan, Singapore
Printed in Hong Kong by Wing King Tong

Contents

Introduction

What do the following people have in common: Julius Caesar, the apostle St. Paul, Dostoyevsky, Vincent van Gogh, the prophet Mohammed, Joan of Arc, the Buddha, Edward Lear, Gustav Flaubert and Alexander the Great? The answer is that they probably all had epilepsy.

Today there are people from all walks of life who suffer from epilepsy, and it is therefore somewhat surprising that any misunderstandings still arise. Indeed, the fear of possible stigmatisation or prejudice results in many people hiding their epilepsy from friends, employers, and sometimes even from members of their own family.

Epilepsy has undoubtedly achieved an unenviable image in people's minds, perhaps largely because of its unpredictable, dramatic and sometimes frightening effects. Although there are many different types of seizures, as will be explained later, it is the convulsion – the falling to the ground, the frothing at the mouth, the flailing of the limbs – that comes to most people's minds when the word epilepsy is mentioned. It is this dramatic event that has always fuelled people's imaginations;

EPILEPSY AMONG THE FAMOUS
Vincent van Gogh, the 19th century Dutch painter, is believed to have suffered from epilepsy.

7

epileptic seizures are mentioned in the earliest Babylonian and Hebrew tracts. In Ancient Greece, at a time obsessed with gods and spirits, Hippocrates was one of the first to try to dispel the mysticism of epileptic seizures. He firmly believed that epilepsy originated in the brain and even went as far as condemning those charlatans who proposed that epilepsy was due to demonic possession.

Yet for the next 2,000 years, it was this theory of demonic possession that led to people with epilepsy being shunned, locked away and subjected to unpleasant, painful and humiliating ordeals in the name of a cure. In the account of the death of the English king, Charles II, there is a description of the treatment of his seizure; this included bleeding him, giving him substances that made him sick, repeated enemas, shaving his head, blistering his skin and then finally forcing an unpleasant concoction down the dying king's throat.

Even as recently as the 19th century, circumcision and castration were proposed as cures of epilepsy. It was not until the end of the 19th century that the first effective drug, potassium bromide, was introduced, and from that time, drug treatment has allowed the majority of people with epilepsy to lead normal, seizure-free lives.

However, there is still, to a certain extent, a stigma attached to what is a common condition (almost every one of us knows someone who has epilepsy, although we may be unaware that he or she does in fact suffer from the condition).

How Many People Suffer from Epilepsy

Out of 50 million people, the approximate population of the UK:

- 1–2.5 million will develop epilepsy in their lifetime.
- 250,000–500,000 will have active epilepsy.
- 10,000–35,000 will develop epilepsy each year.

HOW COMMON IS EPILEPSY?

Epilepsy is extremely common. Each year in the United Kingdom about 25,000 people develop epilepsy, the majority being either children or elderly people (epilepsy infrequently starts between the ages of 20 and 50).

There is about a one in 30 chance of an individual developing epilepsy. However, only one in 200 people has active epilepsy (about 350,000 people in the UK). This implies that most people with epilepsy get better, and indeed this is the case; in about six out of every 10 people the condition resolves itself.

Epilepsy affects males and females almost equally, although certain types of epilepsy are more common in one or other sex. It affects all classes and all races.

Thus epilepsy is extremely common, and usually gets better – this is an important message for all those who develop the condition.

WHO GETS EPILEPSY?
In most people who suffer from epilepsy, the condition begins either in childhood, or after the age of 50.

KEY POINTS

- There are many types of epilepsy and seizures.
- Epilepsy usually begins in childhood or old age.
- Epilepsy is common, but usually resolves itself.

What are seizures and epilepsy?

Seizures, or fits, take many forms. They originate in the brain, and different types of seizures arise in different parts of the brain.

SWEET SENSATIONS
When we smell something, we are activating the temporal lobe of our brain. If this part of the brain becomes damaged then our sense of smell may become impaired.

The brain is involved in forming our emotions, thoughts, memories, in controlling movement and in appreciating sensations, sounds, smells, tastes and sight.

It is divided into two halves joined in the middle; the right half controls the left-hand side of the body and the left half controls the right-hand side.

For most of us, the left half is 'dominant'. In other words, it controls how we form and understand language. Each half (or hemisphere) is further divided into four lobes (see the box opposite).

Damaging one part of the brain will take away its function. For example, damage to the left occipital lobe will result in the person being unable to see anything on the right; damage to the right frontal lobe will cause a

The Structure of the Brain

This view of the left hand side of the brain shows the brain stem, the cerebellum and one of the two cerebral hemispheres. Each hemisphere is composed of four lobes, and each lobe has specific functions.

Outer layer of the cerebral hemisphere is grey matter, consisting of nerve cell bodies

Frontal lobe is involved in conscious thought and movement

White matter is made up of nerve fibres

Parietal lobe is involved in interpreting sensations

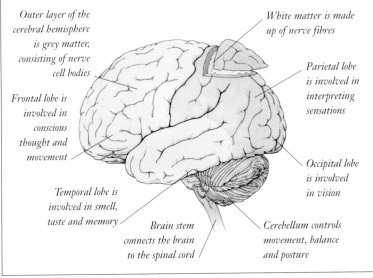

Temporal lobe is involved in smell, taste and memory

Brain stem connects the brain to the spinal cord

Occipital lobe is involved in vision

Cerebellum controls movement, balance and posture

The Lobes of the Brain

Each of the four lobes of each cerebral hemisphere has its own particular physical and mental functions. These can be impaired by brain damage.

FRONTAL LOBE

Among other things, involved in the control of movement.

PARIETAL LOBE

Involved in the appreciation of sensation.

TEMPORAL LOBE

Involved in the appreciation of smells and tastes and the formation of memories.

OCCIPITAL LOBE

Involved in vision.

11

person to be paralysed down the left-hand side. Conversely activating the left occipital lobe, for instance with electrical current, results in the person seeing coloured blobs on the right-hand side, and stimulating over the right frontal lobe causes the left part of the body to move.

A seizure can be likened to an electrical storm. This storm can be confined to one part of the brain, spread to other parts of the brain or involve the whole brain at once. Those that start in one part of the brain are known as 'partial seizures' and those that start in both halves at once are known as 'generalised seizures'. What a person experiences and what is seen by others depend upon where in the brain the seizure starts, and how far and how quickly it spreads.

In the next section we define the different types of seizure in some detail.

ELECTRICAL STORM
An epileptic seizure is like an electrical storm. It can be confined to one part of the brain, it may spread to other parts or it may involve the whole brain.

THE TYPES OF SEIZURE

Almost all seizures are sudden, short-lived and self-limiting. Most occur spontaneously without warning and, as explained above, the form of the seizure depends on the part of the brain involved. Their classification is listed in the table opposite.

PARTIAL SEIZURES

● **Simple partial seizures** These are seizures confined to one small part of the brain, during which there is no loss of consciousness. They are often divided into temporal lobe, frontal lobe, parietal lobe and occipital lobe seizures, depending on where the seizure starts.

In temporal lobe seizures, the patient may experience a feeling of intense fear, vivid memory flashbacks, intense déjà-vu (a feeling of having been in an identical situation before) and unpleasant intense smells or tastes. We can all experience some of these from time to time, and, of course, they are not usually seizures; for example, déjà-vu is a common and normal experience. The main difference is that, with epilepsy, these things happen regularly, without reason, they are short-lived and occur with an intensity that is rare in everyday life.

In frontal lobe seizures, there may be uncontrolled jerking of one arm or leg or the head and eyes may turn to one side.

In parietal lobe seizures, the patient may experience tingling down one side of the body.

In occipital lobe seizures, the patient may experience flashing lights in one half of the vision. The seizure usually lasts a matter of seconds.

- **Complex partial seizures** These are really the next stage up from simple partial seizures, and the clue is in the word 'complex'. In these, the seizure involves a larger part of the brain and spreads to enough of the brain so that the patient is no longer aware of his or her environment (i.e., the patient becomes unconscious). The spread of the seizure can either be so fast that the patient

Classification of Seizures

The broad categories of partial and general seizures can be divided into more specific sub-types.

PARTIAL SEIZURES	A Simple partial seizures
	B Complex partial seizures
	C Secondary generalised seizures

GENERALISED SEIZURES	A Absence seizures (petit mal)
	B Myoclonic seizures
	C Clonic seizures
	D Tonic seizures
	E Tonic-clonic seizures (grand mal)
	F Atonic seizures

13

does not experience the simple partial seizure, or be slow enough for the patient to have, for example, a feeling of déjà-vu, a strange unpleasant taste or an awareness of coloured flashing lights lasting seconds to a few minutes before becoming unaware of the surroundings.

During the seizure, it is quite common for complex, strange or inappropriate actions to occur (these are called 'automatisms'). For example, the patient may fumble with his clothes or make chewing movements.

Occasionally, the actions are coordinated and can even take the form of running, dancing, undressing or speaking nonsense. These seizures usually last a matter of minutes, but are occasionally more prolonged. On coming round, the patient is completely unaware of what he or she has done.

BRAIN ACTIVITY
The orange traces of this coloured EEG show the electrical activity in the brain during an epileptic seizure. During an epileptic seizure, a chaotic and unregulated electrical discharge passes through the brain, causing an abrupt increase in activity.

- **Secondary generalised seizures** These result from the spread of the seizure throughout both halves of the brain; the spread can be slow enough for the patient to have a warning (the aura, which is in fact a simple partial seizure) or so rapid that the patient loses consciousness without an aura. This spread is called secondary generalisation, and the seizure takes the form of a 'generalised tonic-clonic' seizure. In this, the patient often goes stiff (called the tonic phase), and may let out a high-pitched cry; he then falls, may go blue and his arms and legs jerk rhythmically (called the clonic phase), grunting can occur, and he may foam at the mouth.

During the seizure, the patient may bite his tongue or wet himself; it usually lasts a few minutes, and afterwards the patient is often confused, may not know where he is and will often sleep. The after-effects (the 'post-ictal' phase) last for minutes or hours.

This seizure, which used to be called a 'grand mal' attack, is now known as a tonic-clonic seizure, and is also sometimes referred to as a convulsion.

GENERALISED SEIZURES

These are seizures that begin in both halves of the brain at once; as such there is no warning and consciousness is lost immediately. Often this seizure is a tonic-clonic seizure (see above), but it can be a clonic seizure (no stiff phase) or a tonic seizure (no shaking stage, the patient just falls like a board).

There is also a rare type in which the patient just slumps to the ground, but recovers quite quickly (an atonic seizure).

There are also two other categories of generalised seizure: absences and myoclonic jerks.

- **Absence** These used to be called a 'petit mal' attack. They are short blank spells, usually in children, that last just a matter of seconds and can be confused with poor attention or loss of concentration. Children with absence epilepsy can have hundreds of these in a day, and often neither the child nor observers are aware of most of them because they are so brief. They are associated with a particular brain wave pattern that is discussed in the next chapter.

- **Myoclonic seizures** These types of seizure are usually seen in patients with other seizure types, and are very brief jerks of one limb or the whole body. The patient

ABSENCE SEIZURES
The child stares blankly, stops talking and becomes quite unaware during an absence seizure. They usually last only a few seconds.

may describe suddenly dropping a cup of tea as his hand flings up, or his whole body being thrown to the ground.

From these descriptions, it can be seen that there are many different types of seizure, and you are probably already aware that there are other conditions that can be mistaken for a seizure and these will be discussed in the next chapter.

THE CAUSE OF SEIZURE?

All brain activity depends on the passage of electrical signals. The brain consists of millions of cells called neurons, which have bodies and long arms with branches known as axons. It is down these axons that the electrical signals pass, like a telephone signal down a telephone line. When the signal reaches the end of the axon, it causes the release of a chemical; this chemical communicates with a nearby neuron body via special 'receivers' called receptors. These may 'excite' this neuron body, and if the excitation is sufficient, then a further signal is sent (or 'fired') down its axon. This is the way in which the neurons communicate with each other. If only excitation took place in the brain, then eventually all the neurons would be firing together, so causing an 'electrical storm' such as seen in a seizure. But some neurons release a chemical from their axons that inhibits the surrounding neurons, stopping them from 'firing'. The brain functions properly when there is a balance between the excitation and the inhibition. If there is either too much excitation or too little inhibition in a part of the brain (an imbalance), a seizure results.

In partial seizures, the local imbalance between excitation and inhibition can be caused by local damage to the brain, for instance, from lack of oxygen at birth, meningitis or head injuries or by abnormal tissue such as a brain tumour or a defect in brain development.

In some cases, the reasons for the partial seizures are not known.

In generalised seizures, the chemical imbalance affects a wide area of brain, and the brain often shows no obviously abnormal structures. This can be caused by drugs such as cocaine and amphetamines, alterations of the body chemistry, excessive alcohol, inherited or unknown factors. Thus, epileptic seizures are a symptom of an underlying brain disturbance in the same way that stomach ache is a symptom of an underlying gut disturbance (e.g. food poisoning, ulcers, appendicitis, etc.).

How Nerve Signals are Transmitted

Electrical signals are carried along a nerve cell via its axon. For a signal to cross the synapse (gap) between two nerve cells, chemical neurotransmitters must pass from the synaptic knob to receptors on the next cell.

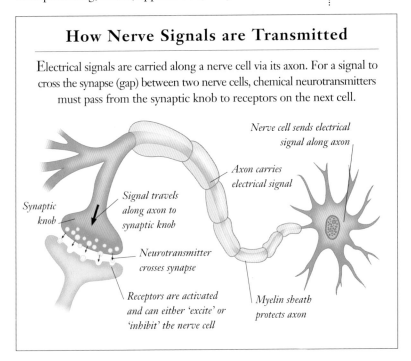

Nerve cell sends electrical signal along axon

Axon carries electrical signal

Signal travels along axon to synaptic knob

Synaptic knob

Neurotransmitter crosses synapse

Receptors are activated and can either 'excite' or 'inhibit' the nerve cell

Myelin sheath protects axon

17

EPILEPSY?

Epilepsy is defined as a condition in which the person is prone to recurrent epileptic seizures, so diagnosis is a measure of the probability of having epileptic seizures. If you have one seizure brought on by excessive alcohol, and then you become teetotal, the chances of having another seizure are very small and you would not be diagnosed as having epilepsy. If, on the other hand, you had a number of seizures because of a damaged part of your brain, the chances of having another seizure are very high, and you would be diagnosed as having epilepsy.

The decision about whether a patient does, or does not, have epilepsy is not always clear cut. We all have a lifetime chance of having a seizure of about one in 30 (29 to 1 against for those who bet, i.e. 'an outside chance'), and we can considerably increase our chances of having a seizure by drinking excessively or taking certain drugs. Most doctors only diagnose patients as having epilepsy if they have two seizures within a year, because, in this instance, the chances of having a third seizure are probably over 80% (4 to 1 on, or in other words 'a sure thing').

The difficulty arises in patients who have had just one seizure. In this instance, the doctor usually assesses what the chances of having another seizure are, aided and abetted by various investigations, and by knowledge of the type of seizure and the probable cause.

Most doctors in the United Kingdom do not usually treat one single seizure because of the low odds of having another seizure (less than 50/50), and the possible side-effects of medication.

ALCOHOL AND SEIZURES
Excessive alcohol, or withdrawal from alcohol, can cause seizures, but not necessarily epilepsy.

The second difficult question is, if a patient is diagnosed as having epilepsy, how many seizure-free years must pass before he is no longer thought to have epilepsy? Unfortunately, there is no simple answer to this question, but it is certainly true that most people with epilepsy eventually stop having seizures, and thus should not be registered as having epilepsy (if someone has not had a headache for 10 years, it would be perverse to call him a headache sufferer).

It is important to bear in mind that epilepsy is a symptom and not a disease as such. A symptom is something experienced by patients, indicative of an underlying disease. This is the case with epilepsy, which should be considered as an indicator of some underlying brain problem. A wide spectrum of brain conditions can result in epilepsy.

WHAT IS AN EPILEPSY SYNDROME?

A syndrome is a medical term referring to a specific condition in which characteristic groups of symptoms occur together. They are often named after the person who first described them.

For example, West's Syndrome is characterised by infantile spasms (the baby suddenly bends over) with a particular brain wave pattern, and often with mental handicap, in babies aged between 3–12 months. Most of these children will go on to have epilepsy that is difficult to treat and mental handicap. This explains what occurs and what happens, but does not tell us the underlying cause of the seizures (there are, in fact, a multitude of causes of West's Syndrome).

The most common epilepsy syndromes are benign childhood epilepsy, with distinctive changes on the

Features of Epilepsy Syndromes

The two most commonly found types of epilepsy syndrome are benign childhood epilepsy and primary generalised epilepsy.

EPILEPSY SYNDROME	FEATURES
Benign childhood epilepsy with distinctive EEG changes	• Occurs between 2 and 14 years of age. • Can be inherited. • Seizures involve face, throat and tongue, and consciousness is preserved. • Occasionally tonic-clonic seizures occur during sleep. • Typical EEG pattern. • Most get completely better and drug treatment is not usually necessary.
Primary generalised epilepsy	• Usually occurs in childhood or adolescence. • Can be divided into many different syndromes. • Can be inherited. • Seizure types consist of a combination of absences, tonic-clonic seizures and myoclonic seizures. • Seizures usually occur on, or within a couple of hours of, waking. • Typical EEG pattern. • Usually well controlled with valproate.

EEG, and primary generalised, or generalised, epilepsies. The table opposite outlines the features that characterise these two epilepsy syndromes.

KEY POINTS

- Seizures in different parts of the brain produce different effects.
- Seizures take many forms and can be likened to electrical storms in the brain.

Diagnosis of epilepsy

When a doctor first sees a patient whose symptoms suggest a possible diagnosis of epilepsy, there are two questions that need to be addressed. First, does the patient definitely have epileptic seizures, and secondly, if the seizures are epileptic, what is the cause of the epilepsy?

IS IT EPILEPSY?

Many conditions can be confused with epileptic seizures. In adults, the most common are syncope (fainting), migraine, hyperventilation and panic attacks and 'pseudo-seizures'. In children, other conditions that can also commonly be confused with epilepsy include breath-holding attacks and night terrors.

SYNCOPE

Syncope is the medical term for fainting, and occurs when not enough blood gets to the brain. The most common mechanism of syncope is the classic swoon (the

FEELING FAINT
A person on the point of fainting may feel hot, dizzy and sick. Sometimes a classic faint is confused with an epileptic seizure, as jerking may be present in both states.

'vasovagal' attack), in response to, for instance, seeing something unpleasant, experiencing excruciating pain or standing for a long period of time in a hot enclosed space. Occasionally, syncope is due to a heart disturbance (for example, if the heart goes into an abnormal rhythm), or it can be precipitated by particular events (including coughing or urinating).

The classic faint is well known to all of us; the person feels dizzy, hot and sick, becomes very pale (a deathly white), his or her vision goes grey and then he or she slumps to the ground. At this point, the blood flow to the brain increases and the person comes round quite quickly. At first sight, it would seem difficult to confuse this with the seizures mentioned in the previous chapter. However, some jerking of the limbs can occur, especially if the person is propped up, because this may prevent enough blood reaching the brain. The jerking is occasionally prolonged, but seldom has the coordinated pattern of a tonic-clonic seizure. In some partial seizures, the person may experience similar feelings to those of a faint so that the two conditions are not always easy to distinguish.

MIGRAINE

As most people are aware, migraines often begin with a disturbance in vision or can be associated with tingling in the arm or face, and rarely with a disturbance of speech. It can be difficult to distinguish this from a simple partial seizure, especially because it is not uncommon to have a splitting headache after a seizure. Consciousness is, however, practically never lost with a migraine. There are also differences in the disturbance of vision between that in migraine and that in epilepsy. Disturbances of vision in migraine usually evolve over minutes, and have a simple form (e.g. circles of light or bright dots); disturbances in vision in epilepsy evolve more rapidly over seconds and are usually more complex (e.g. multi-coloured shapes or sometimes scenes or faces). In addition, if tingling is experienced, it tends to spread slowly up the arm in migraine and rapidly in seizures. In most cases, there is little doubt about whether an attack is caused by migraine or epilepsy, but occasionally it can present a diagnostic puzzle.

HYPERVENTILATION AND PANIC ATTACKS

Overbreathing (hyperventilation) is not uncommon, especially in those under a lot of stress, or in those who tend to panic ('panic attacks'). The immediate feeling is usually described as a sudden difficulty in catching one's breath, and a feeling of panic (although these do not always have to be present). During overbreathing, a person breathes out too much carbon dioxide, and when this happens the acidity of the blood changes. This affects nerve activity, and can cause tingling sensations, spasms of the hand, lightheadedness and even black-outs. These attacks are best treated with relaxation and breathing exercises. Rebreathing into a paper bag during an attack enables a person to rebreathe the carbon dioxide that he is breathing out and, therefore, prevent or reverse the unpleasant effects of hyperventilation.

CONTROLLING BREATHING
Breathing into a paper bag during hyperventilation will cause carbon dioxide to be reinhaled, restore the level of acidity in the blood and thereby calm breathing.

'PSEUDOSEIZURES'

These are often the most difficult to distinguish from true epileptic seizures. These attacks are 'all in the mind', although usually involuntary and occurring without any conscious motivation. Occasionally these attacks are 'put on', but for the most part the patient has little control and they can be likened to an emotional outburst. The patient may fall, appear to lose consciousness and then thrash around or lie motionless. These attacks often have some deep-rooted emotional basis, and may require psychiatric treatment. They do not respond to drugs for epilepsy. When it is difficult to tell these from an epileptic seizure, patients are admitted to hospital for close observation.

BREATH-HOLDING ATTACKS

Unfortunately toddlers can hold their breath until they turn blue, and may resort to this if they do not get their own way. Usually the attack stops there, but occasionally a strong-willed toddler can hold his breath until he passes out. These do not require drug treatment, and the attacks usually stop of their own accord.

NIGHT TERRORS

These affect children usually under the age of five years. A few hours after falling asleep, the child appears to wake, is terrified and cannot be comforted. In the morning the child usually has no memory of the night's events.

Although worrying, these are completely innocent and do not require treatment.

DIAGNOSING THE PROBLEM

The most important diagnostic tool is the 'medical history', the question and answer session that occurs between a patient and his or her doctor in the consulting room or surgery. The doctor will try to determine whether the episodes are seizures by asking for a detailed description of what happens, and obviously, as consciousness may be impaired, it is important that there is someone present who has seen an episode in order to help with the description (or even better a video of the episode).

The doctor will be interested in what the underlying cause of the seizures is and will thus ask questions about head injuries, problems with birth, whether the patient has had meningitis, alcohol consumption and whether other people in the family have epilepsy. He will also be interested in the impact that epilepsy will have on the patient's life, and so will ask about the patient's job and home life. Lastly, he will examine the patient, looking for clues as to whether there is some underlying brain abnormality, and may also check the heart, especially if syncope is suspected.

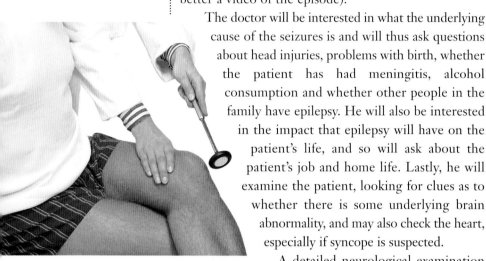

TESTING REFLEXES
Leg reflexes form part of the detailed neurological examination that your doctor will carry out to help him or her diagnose the cause of your seizures.

A detailed neurological examination involves checking the eyes, the face, coordination, power and sensation in the limbs, and the reflexes in the arms, legs and feet. Besides blood and other routine tests, there are three special investigations that the doctor may decide to request that we will describe in some detail – electroencephalography (EEG), computed tomography (CT) scanning and magnetic resonance imaging (MRI).

ELECTROENCEPHALOGRAPHY (EEG)

This is literally 'recording the electricity from the brain'. Wires are attached to different parts of the head which are then connected to an amplifier; this amplifier magnifies the small electrical signal from the brain and records this signal onto paper. EEG is merely a recording of the internal electrical patterns of the brain, and as such does not involve the passage of any electricity into or out of the brain. It is thus a harmless and painless investigation, and is of great use to the doctor.

Normally, the tracing shows a wave pattern (the 'brain waves'), with one wave occurring every tenth of a second or so. The waves slow down during sleep, and speed up when the patient is alert. If the patient is prone to epilepsy, the electrical pattern may be different, in particular showing what are called spikes or spike/wave patterns. Spikes can be picked up by an EEG performed in between seizures in about half the patients with epilepsy, but, if spikes are present, there is a 99% chance of the person having epilepsy. EEGs are occasionally performed during sleep because spikes are more likely to be picked up during this period.

A particular EEG pattern, called 3 per second spike and wave, is of particular importance. This is seen in patients with absence epilepsy, which requires a specific form of drug treatment and has a good outcome.

EEGs performed during a seizure, and especially if the patient is videoed at the same time, are of great use in patients in whom the diagnosis is in some doubt and in identifying exactly where the seizure starts (necessary, for instance, in assessing patients for epilepsy surgery). One such test is called video telemetry. This involves patients being admitted to hospital for several days during which they are constantly monitored by EEG and video. Sometimes it is also necessary to reduce or withdraw the patient's antiepileptic drugs to induce a seizure while the patient is being monitored.

CT SCANNING

Computed tomography, or CT, is literally the use of a computer to give detailed pictures of 'slices' of the brain. This diagnostic technique uses X-rays; however, unlike a conventional skull X-ray in which X-rays are fired at one side of the head, with a photographic plate on the other side, in a CT scan, X-rays are fired at different angles and picked up by 'receivers'. The information obtained is then analysed by a computer that displays the X-ray signal as a series of pictures of slices through the skull and brain, something like slices through a loaf of bread.

By using this technique, it is now possible to demonstrate such brain abnormalities as tumours, strokes, brain haemorrhages or Alzheimer's disease. However, CT is gradually being replaced by magnetic resonance imaging or MRI (see below) in the diagnosis of the causes of epilepsy. This is because MRI is a much more sensitive test and gives much clearer pictures.

SEEING INSIDE THE BRAIN
CT scanning uses X-rays to create slice images through regions of the body. This coloured scan shows a section through a normal brain.

During a CT scan, the patient has to lie with his or her head stationary in the scanner for a number of minutes. This is an entirely painless procedure.

Occasionally a dye is injected into a vein in the arm to highlight certain parts of the brain in order to gain more information from the scan.

MAGNETIC RESONANCE IMAGING (MRI)

This procedure does not use X-rays at all. A large, powerful magnet is placed around the patient's head. The atoms in the brain orient themselves along this magnetic field. A burst of radio waves is then 'fired' at the patient and the hydrogen atoms in the brain wobble (resonate). As the hydrogen atoms gradually return to rest, they give off radio waves that are picked up by 'receivers' and analysed by a computer; this gives detailed pictures of the brain. This technique is very safe and entirely painless; however, it does involve lying in the scanner, which is an enclosed space, for some time (usually 10–20 minutes), which some people find unpleasant. Also, because powerful magnets are used, people with some types of metal implants (for instance, clips or wires from previous brain or other operations and pacemakers) cannot be scanned.

This technique can detect many subtle and small abnormalities that were previously undetectable by CT scanning. As MRI techniques improve so the underlying cause of epilepsy is being discovered in more and more patients. MRI is especially useful in assessing the suitability of patients who have not responded to drugs for surgical treatment (see p.47). Also, using computer analysis, the relative size of different brain structures can be calculated. This is important in, for instance, analysing certain areas of the brain (especially an area known as the hippocampus) that, when damaged, can cause seizures.

MRI BRAIN SCAN
This false-colour MRI scan shows a cross-section through a normal brain. MRI is increasingly being used to detect brain abnormalities.

THE CAUSES OF EPILEPSY

As has been emphasised, epilepsy is a symptom and not a disease. There are many causes such as infections, head

Causes of Epilepsy from Birth to Old Age

This chart lists the likely causes of epilepsy in both children and adults. Birth trauma and genetic disease may cause childhood epilepsy, while in adults brain tumours or stokes are common causes.

- Inherited brain diseases, e.g, tuberous sclerosis.
- Inherited epilepsies, e.g., primary generalised epilepsy.
- Birth trauma.
- Febrile convulsions.
- Brain infections, e.g., meningitis, encephalitis, brain abscesses.
- Recreational drugs and alcohol, e.g., cocaine, amphetamines, 'Ecstasy'.

- Head trauma.
- Blood chemical abnormalities, e.g., low calcium, magnesium or glucose.
- Cerebral haemorrhages.
- Brain tumours, e.g., gliomas, meningiomas.
- Strokes.
- Dementia, e.g., Alzheimer's disease.

injuries, brain tumours, brain injuries at birth and inherited diseases (see above). Occasionally epilepsy can present many years after the damage has occurred. For example, it is not uncommon for people who have sustained a brain injury in childhood to present with epilepsy in their 20s.

For many sufferers (about 70 per cent), no known cause is ever found. In the generalised epilepsies, genetic factors are likely play a role, and some epilepsies are hereditary, but in most cases this is not so (how, for example, do you inherit a head injury?). Except in a few genetically inherited conditions that can cause epilepsy, the risks of passing the epilepsy on to your offspring are very small indeed.

KEY POINTS

- Many conditions are confused with epilepsy, the most common being fainting, migraine, panic attacks, 'pseudoseizures', breath-holding attacks and night terrors (the last two in children).
- Epilepsy can be caused by infections, head injuries, brain tumours, brain injuries at birth and inherited diseases, but often the cause is not known.
- Investigations for diagnosing epilepsy include EEG, CT scan and MRI, but the patient's medical history is of greatest importance in making the diagnosis.
- Risks of passing epilepsy on to offspring are very small.

Treatment of epilepsy

Much can be done to prevent a person coming to any great harm during an epileptic attack by following a few simple procedures. Drug therapy can help to cut down the number of such attacks.

FIRST AID TREATMENT
Although a major seizure is frightening to watch, stay calm and loosen any tight clothing to ensure that the person can breathe.

MANAGING CONVULSIONS

Seizures and convulsions are often frightening to watch, especially because the person may turn blue, have wild, jerking movements, foam at the mouth and cry out. People often wish to intervene by placing an object in the person's mouth to 'prevent him swallowing his tongue'

What to Do During a Convulsion

There are a few simple procedures that should be followed if you are present during a seizure. The most important thing is to stay calm and let the seizure run its course.

- During a convulsion the patient should be laid on the ground away from objects that can cause injury, the head should be cushioned and the patient should not be restrained in any way.
- After the convulsion, the patient should be turned on to his left side, in the recovery position, and someone should remain with the patient until he is fully recovered.
- Sometimes, confusion can mimic aggression. In these cases the patient should not be restrained, but gently coaxed out of danger. At this stage, if anything is blocking the airway, it should be cleared.
- If the convulsion lasts longer than 5 minutes, or if the patient is having repeated convulsions without consciousness being regained, then call an ambulance.

and by calling an ambulance. The former intervention can, however, be dangerous; objects should not be placed in the patient's mouth during the convulsion, because the patient may bite the hand of the helper and bite the object resulting in damage to the teeth and mouth.

If you are experiencing a lot of seizures, having someone call an ambulance every time is embarrassing and usually quite unnecessary.

The chart at the top of this page shows the correct procedure in the event of a seizure.

Some patients have recurrent prolonged seizures, and occasionally carers will be asked to give these patients a drug called diazepam, either by mouth or as a suppository,

THE RECOVERY POSITION
To place someone in the recovery position, gently pull the person towards you with one hand on the lower part of the body. Protect the patient's face with the other hand.

in order to stop the seizure. This policy should be discussed with the doctor in charge of the care of any patient who has repeated episodes of seizures lasting longer than 20–30 minutes, because immediate drug therapy may be beneficial to the patient and prevent the patient needing to go to hospital.

LONG-TERM TREATMENT

The aim of long-term treatment is to stop all seizures, and this can be attained in most (about 80 per cent) patients. The following are the three main ways to achieve this:

- Avoiding those things that cause seizures.
- Drug treatment.
- Brain surgery.

Very occasionally, patients who have warnings that last a long time before losing consciousness are able to control their seizure and prevent the loss of consciousness. This is sometimes achieved by intense concentration during the warning period.

AVOIDING TRIGGERS

In many patients, avoiding certain factors will lessen the frequency of seizures and in a few will prevent them altogether. Very rarely, people can have seizures brought on by hearing particular pieces of music, reading, hot showers, seeing certain patterns, etc., and these are referred to as 'reflex epilepsies'. For most, however, no specific trigger is ever noticed. There are nevertheless four things that can induce or worsen seizures in many – excessive alcohol, lack of sleep, stress and fever. Lastly, a few patients are sensitive to flashing lights (this is called photosensitivity (see p.36).

TRIGGER FACTORS
Very raely, certain types of music can trigger an epileptic seizure in susceptible people.

ALCOHOL AND SLEEP DEPRIVATION

Often patients who have primary generalised epilepsies are particularly susceptible to seizures following binges of alcohol or sleep deprivation, but these are almost certainly two factors that all people with epilepsy should try to avoid. Indeed, alcohol abuse or suddenly stopping a pattern of alcohol abuse can induce seizures in almost anyone, and seizures are thus a common complication of alcoholism. For those whose seizures are particularly exacerbated by sleep deprivation, getting tired, missing sleep and sometimes shift work are inadvisable.

SLEEP DEPRIVATION
Many find that a lack of sleep will prompt a seizure. People with epilepsy should ensure that they get regular and sufficient sleep.

STRESS

Although it is often difficult to identify the effects of stress, it can nevertheless have a profound effect upon seizure control. Furthermore, relaxation exercises, stress management and such therapies as aromatherapy can have a beneficial effect, and thus should be recommended to many patients. Often, counselling those who have difficulties coping with their epilepsy can help seizure control. Depression, low mood and low moral can also increase the frequency of seizures. These factors can in addition affect how regularly patients take their medication (compliance), and thus indirectly worsen seizure control.

FEVER AND HIGH TEMPERATURES

During any illness seizures can get worse, and this is especially so in young children if a fever is present. This is because a high body temperature makes the brain more likely to have a seizure. Thus, at the first signs of a fever, the body temperature should be kept down with regular paracetamol and, if necessary, a fan or cold sponging. Another instance in which the body temperature can rise resulting in increased seizure frequency is sunstroke, which is usually due to a combination of excessive sun exposure and dehydration.

PHOTOSENSITIVITY

Recently much has been made of light sensitivity (photosensitivity) and the relationship of seizures to video games, televisions or computer screen; in fact, less than five per cent of all people with epilepsy are sensitive to flashing lights. The photosensitive seizures usually occur with lights that flicker from 5–30 times per second and television and video games (both of which have flickering screens) can induce photosensitive seizures in susceptible individuals. However, children in the UK spend a large amount of time watching television and playing video games, and thus any seizure that occurs during this time may be purely coincidental.

Other common triggers include:

- Sunlight reflecting off water.
- Passing a line of trees through which the sun is shining.
- Stroboscopic lights (although local authorities do have guidelines on the flash rate of strobe lighting, it is perhaps best avoided by susceptible individuals).

In some patients with photosensitivity, avoidance of what triggers their seizures or taking certain precautions, such as the use of sunglasses in bright light, rather than antiepileptic drug treatment, may be all that they need to do to prevent the seizures.

The following are the precautions that can be taken to avoid television-induced seizures for those not on drugs:

- Viewing the television in a well-lit room.
- Viewing the television from an angle.
- Sitting at least 2.5 metres from the television set.
- Changing channels with a remote control rather than getting too close to the screen.
- Covering one eye and/or using high-frequency (100 Hz) televisions.

Seizures are rarely triggered by cinema films, and usually computer screens operate at a high frequency to avoid provoking seizures. However, in both these instances, the content, if it consists of a changing geometric pattern at the correct frequency, can very occasionally provoke a seizure. Antiepileptic drug treatment is usually effective in preventing photosensitive seizures.

DRUG TREATMENT

Since the earliest times, people have been seeking effective drugs for epilepsy, and through the ages such cures as powdered human skull, vultures' blood and mistletoe have all been tried. The first effective therapy, however, was reported in 1857 by Sir Charles Locock, an obstetrician, who had an interest in epilepsy because of the mistaken idea, common at that time, that in some women epilepsy came from their wombs. The drug he used was potassium bromide, and this remained the most effective therapy for epilepsy until 1912, when phenobarbitone was introduced.

The main problems with bromides are their unacceptable side -effects. In fact the play-off of side-effects against the effectiveness of an antiepileptic drug is still at the heart of antiepileptic drug treatment.

EARLY TREATMENT
Medication using the mistletoe plant was among the earliest attempts to treat people suffering from epilepsy.

HOW IS THE DRUG ABSORBED

Once swallowed an antiepileptic drug is absorbed into the bloodstream, passing into the brain, which is where the drug acts. Whether an antiepileptic drug is taken on an empty or a full stomach can affect the amount of drug absorbed; they should generally be taken at the same time in relation to meals. Once the drug has passed around the bloodstream, it is removed from the body, either being broken down (metabolised) by the liver or filtered out by the kidneys and passed out in the urine (different drugs are removed in different ways). If a drug is removed from the body very quickly, then it has to be taken frequently (3–4 times a day) to keep the blood levels reasonably high; conversely if a drug is only removed slowly then it can be taken once a day.

WHICH DRUG?
Your doctor will choose an antiepileptic drug appropriate to your type of epilepsy and your needs.

HOW DO THESE DRUGS WORK?

It is not certain exactly how most antiepileptic drugs work, but there do seem to be a number of important mechanisms. In an earlier chapter (see pp.17–18), it was explained that seizures may result when the excitation and inhibition occurring in the brain are not balanced. Some antiepileptic drugs correct this chemical imbalance. Others work in a different fashion, by 'stabilising' neurons, and thus preventing excessive firing of axons.

THE RIGHT DRUG FOR THE PATIENT

Most antiepileptic drugs work in different types of epilepsy, and often it is just a matter of choosing the drug that suits the patient best. Interestingly, what may be a very effective drug in one patient may be useless in another. However, some antiepileptic drugs only work in particular forms of epilepsy (e.g. ethosuximide for absence epilepsy) and, indeed, some antiepileptic drugs can make some forms of epilepsy worse (e.g. carbamazepine for myoclonic seizures). A list of the drugs that are used most often in particular seizure types is presented in the table on the next page.

SIDE-EFFECTS

There are three main types of side-effects of antiepileptic drugs. These are: dose-related side-effects, individual or idiosyncratic side-effects and chronic side-effects.

● **Dose-related side-effects** These are seen in all patients if the dose of the antiepileptic drug is high enough (this is sometimes called drug intoxication). The amount of drug that can be tolerated varies from patient to patient. With most of the antiepileptic drugs, dizziness, double vision, unsteadiness, drowsiness and headache are the most common dose-related side-effects. They are alleviated by reducing the dose of the drug, but in the case of drugs that are removed slowly from the body, it may take several days for the effects of this to be felt. Importantly, many people become used to some immediate side effects (especially drowsiness) after being on a drug for a little while, and thus it is always prudent to give a drug a month or so before abandoning it because of mild side-effects. Most of the antiepileptic drugs can also interfere with concentration and intellectual ability.

● **Idiosyncratic side-effects** These are those that only occur in some people and are essentially allergies. They take the form of rashes or various blood disorders. As they do not depend on the dose of the drug, the only way to overcome these side-effects is to discontinue the drug.

Types of Seizure and Appropriate Drug Treatments

Some anticonvulsant drugs only work for particular forms of epilepsy, and it is important to choose the right drug to suit the patient and the type of seizures being experienced.

SEIZURE TYPE	DRUGS TRIED FIRST	OTHER DRUGS THAT ARE USED	
PARTIAL SEIZURES			
Simple partial	Carbamazepine	Acetazolamide	Vigabatrin
Complex partial	Phenytoin	Clobazam	Tiagabine
Secondary generalised	Valproate	Gabapentin	
		Lamotrigine	
		Phenobarbitone	
		Primidone	
GENERALISED SEIZURES			
Absences	Ethosuximide	Acetazolamide	Lamotrigine
	Valproate	Clonazepam	
Atonic/Tonic	Valproate	Acetazolamide	Lamotrigine
		Carbamazepine	Phenobarbitone
		Clobazam	Primidone
		Clonazepam	Phenytoin
		Gabapentin	Topiramate
Tonic-clonic/Clonic	Carbamazepine	Acetazolamide	Primidone
	Phenytoin	Lamotrigine	Topiramate
	Valproate	Phenobarbitone	Vigabatrin
Myoclonic	Clonazepam	Acetazolamide	Primidone
	Valproate	Phenobarbitone	Piracetam

- **Chronic side-effects** These are the ones that occur after taking the drug for many years. The chronic side-effects of the newer antiepileptic drugs are thus not as well documented as the chronic side-effects of the older, more established drugs. The table on p. 42 includes the more common side-effects that can occur with some antiepileptic drugs.

DRUGS INTERACTIONS

The blood levels of antiepileptic drugs can be affected by other drugs (including other antiepileptic drugs), resulting in either a fall in the blood level (causing seizures), or a rise in the blood level (causing side effects). This is because the break down, excretion and absorption of antiepileptic drugs can be affected by other drugs. It is thus important to check before taking any other medication, including those that can be bought without a prescription (see table on p.43 for a list of some of the commonly prescribed drugs that interact with antiepileptic drugs). When a new antiepileptic drug is added to a patient's antiepileptic drug treatment, it is often necessary to change the dose of the existing antiepileptic drugs and to monitor blood levels.

ADJUSTING THE DOSAGE
Side-effects, such as headache and dizziness, are a problem for some people and may mean that the dosage needs adjusting.

Antiepileptic drugs can also affect the blood levels of other drugs. This is important for the contraceptive pill, because many antiepileptic drugs increase the body's ability to break down the pill, rendering it ineffective. In this instance, higher doses of the pill are required. Breakthrough bleeding is a sign that the dose of the pill is probably not high enough, and that it will not be providing adequate contraception. A similar increase in drug

41

Possible Side-effects of Antiepileptic Drugs

Antiepileptic drugs can produce three main types of side-effect – dose-related, individual or idiosyncratic (rare allergic reactions), and chronic.

DOSE-RELATED	IDIOSYNCRATIC	CHRONIC
Double vision	Rash	Weight gain
Unsteadiness	Blood disorders	Vitamin deficiencies
Dizziness	Liver failure	Changes in facial
Sleepiness	Psychosis/depression	appearance
Headache		Acne
Stomach upset		Mood changes
Slowness		Sedation

metabolism occurs when antiepileptic drugs are combined with warfarin (a drug for preventing blood clotting), and this may result in the need for larger doses of warfarin.

STARTING AND STOPPING MEDICATION

Starting antiepileptic drugs at a high dose can result in side-effects being experienced. Antiepileptic drugs should therefore be introduced cautiously and the dose increased in gradual steps. The final dose is determined by the balance between seizure control and side-effects.

It is important to realise that individual patients require different doses and that the final dose may be even more than the generally recommended maximum dose for the drug. In this instance, there is usually no need for concern if the patient is not experiencing side-effects. If a drug does not work or if the side-effects are unacceptable, another drug is tried. Most patients are controlled on only one antiepileptic drug (known as monotherapy, literally one therapy). In a smaller number of patients, two or more different antiepileptic drugs are necessary (this is known as polytherapy, which literally means many therapies).

For the following reasons the doctor will try, wherever possible, to avoid polytherapy:

- Some antiepileptic drugs interact with other anti-epileptic drugs.
- Side-effects are often greater in polytherapy.
- It is difficult to remember to take many different drugs and thus compliance is worse.
- There is a greater potential for mistakes.

When a drug is being stopped, the dose must be decreased in gradual steps. A flurry of bad seizures can result from stopping an antiepileptic drug suddenly, even if the drug had not apparently been effective.

Substances that Interact with Antiepileptic Drugs

Below is a list of the commonly prescribed substances that interact with antiepileptic medication.

SUBSTANCE	FUNCTION
Allopurinol	Gout
Aminophylline	Asthma
Amiodarone	Heart rhythm disturbances
Antacids	Indigestion
Aspirin	Pain killer
Cimetidine	Indigestion, peptic ulcers
Co-proxamol	Pain killer
Diltiazem	Angina
Erythromycin	Antibiotic
Fluoxetine	Antidepressant
Folic acid	Vitamin
Imipramine	Antidepressant
Omeprazole	Indigestion, peptic ulcers
Co-trimoxazole	Antibiotic
Verapamil	Angina

TAKING DRUGS REGULARLY

The taking of a drug according to instructions received is known as compliance. Poor compliance (that is, failure to take a drug as instructed – either not taking the drug at all or taking it irregularly) is a major cause of the failure of antiepileptic drug treatment.

As it usually takes some time (days or weeks) for an antiepileptic drug to be fully effective, and seizure occurrence is usually unpredictable, it is imperative to take the drug regularly in order to prevent seizures. When patients are not having seizures they feel perfectly well (apart from the side-effects of the antiepileptic drugs), and so it is thus not surprising that the occasional dose is missed either consciously or subconsciously.

Following a Regular Routine

It is also very easy for patients on regular medication to forget whether or not the last dose was taken. It is important for patients to build up a regular routine of drug taking. Compliance is not helped if a drug has to be taken more than twice a day, especially in children who are not keen to take drugs midday at school. The situation becomes even worse if the patient is on polytherapy. A drug wallet, with the tablets divided into different compartments according to the time of day and the day of the week, is often very useful. All that then needs to be done is for the compartments in the wallet to be replenished each week. Drug wallets are also useful for those who have poor memories or very busy routines.

Stopping Suddenly

Occasionally patients decide to stop their drugs suddenly (often because of depression or low morale). This is potentially dangerous because it can lead to prolonged and frequent seizures. Also, during periods of vomiting or diarrhoea, the tablets may not be absorbed, and in these cases the tablets should be retaken or antisickness (antiemetic) drugs prescribed by the doctor; on occasion admission to hospital is necessary.

MEDICATION ORGANISER
There are various devices available on the market to help you to take the right pill at the right time of day.

TAKING THE RIGHT DOSE

Last of all, misunderstandings between doctors and patients can lead to the wrong dosages being taken. After any consultation it is important to be clear precisely how much of each drug needs to be taken; if necessary the doctor should write this information down. When coming for appointments, it is usually a good idea for patients to bring their drug with them. Answers to vague enquiries about drugs are rarely helpful. For example, it would be impossible to give a response to 'Well, I take two blue or is it red pills in the morning, and then a white. No, I take the white pill in the evening'.

MONITORING THE DRUGS

It is important to monitor the effectiveness of an antiepileptic drug, and the best method is by seizure frequency. It is often surprisingly difficult to remember exactly how many seizures have occurred and thus a written record is mandatory for patients who have frequent seizures. This seizure diary can then be reviewed at each appointment with the doctor. It is important for patients to learn to differentiate between their different seizure types, and to record the frequency of each of them separately. Information of when antiepileptic drugs were started should also be included.

KEEPING A DIARY
Keep a note of any seizures and, if relevant, any obvious triggers. This will help your doctor to determine the effectiveness of your antiepileptic medication.

The most important guide to dosage is how well the seizures are controlled and how well or unwell a patient feels. However, occasionally it is helpful to take a blood sample (usually before the morning dose, although this is not always practical) in order to work out the blood levels of an antiepileptic drug. Much is made of blood levels,

45

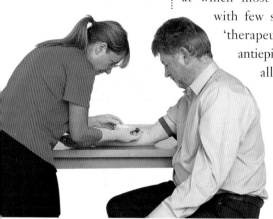

but it is important to keep these in context. The levels at which most patients have good seizure control with few side-effects give rise to the so-called 'therapeutic range' of blood levels for some antiepileptic drugs. The problem is that we are all individuals and what is an effective blood level for most people may be too high or too low for a minority. Blood levels can, however, give the doctor a rough idea of whether the dose of a drug is adequate or not.

There are also other circumstances in which blood levels are very useful:

- If poor seizure control occurs

BLOOD LEVELS
A simple blood test is used to measure the levels of antiepileptic medication in your blood. This can help your GP to determine whether the dosage of the drug is correct.

(blood levels may have fallen).

- To check for compliance.
- If other drugs (including other antiepileptic drugs) that can interfere with the antiepileptic drug therapy are started.
- During pregnancy and illness when drug levels may change.
- In patients with severe learning difficulties, who may not be able to communicate whether or not they are experiencing side-effects.

The following chapter will describe the various drugs available for treatment of epilepsy individually.

SURGERY FOR EPILEPSY

It has been estimated that about 12,500 patients with epilepsy in the UK could benefit from epilepsy surgery. The potential for using surgery, and its success, may increase as the technique called magnetic resonance imaging (MRI – see pp.28–29) improves and the cause of seizures can be identified in more and more patients.

Epilepsy surgery is a major undertaking, because it involves removing the part of the brain where the seizures begin and obviously this is not without risk. Epilepsy surgery is therefore reserved for those patients whose seizures are resistant to drug treatment (also known as 'drug resistant', 'refractory' or 'pharmacoresistant' patients) and in whom there is little chance of the seizures improving.

MANY COULD BENEFIT
Thousands of epilepsy sufferers could be helped by surgery, and it is likely to be more widely used as techniques are developed to identify the exact cause of seizures.

CRITERIA

Even before investigating a patient for epilepsy surgery, several other criteria have to be fulfilled:

• It has to be felt that the seizures are one of the main causes of a patient's disability (a severely handicapped patient may have uncontrolled seizures that are only a minor problem compared with the rest of his or her disability problems).

• Similarly, it has to be felt by both the doctor and the patient that stopping the seizures would result in a significant improvement in the quality of life (undertaking brain surgery for instance in someone who is suicidal or severely depressed for reasons other than their epilepsy or in whom the epilepsy is only of small consequence is obviously not to be recommended).

• The patient must be able to understand the possible risks and benefits of the epilepsy surgery.

TESTS BEFORE SURGERY

There are then several tests that have to be performed before the decision to opt for surgery is taken:

• **Brain imaging** by MRI is used in order to identify any brain abnormalities that may be the cause of the epilepsy.

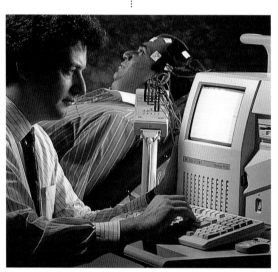

If no such abnormality can be detected, this does not preclude epilepsy surgery, but makes it far less likely to be successful and it will rarely be worth pursuing.

• **Psychological testing** is usually carried out in some detail. This usually involves a number of word, memory and drawing/constructing tests that will elucidate the functioning of different parts of a person's brain.

MONITORING THE BRAIN
By attaching small electrodes to the patient's scalp, a doctor can use an EEG machine to monitor brain activity. The patient's brain waves are displayed on the screen.

This kind of testing is performed in order to identify whether any psychological problem or condition present is related to the part of the brain causing the seizures, the importance of this part of the brain for a patient's memory, speech, etc., and lastly as a baseline for comparison with psychology after surgery has taken place.

• **The measurement of the brain waves** by EEG (electroencephalography) also plays a pivotal role. Usually this involves a technique in which the brain waves are correlated with a video of the seizure in order to identify where the seizure starts. This is necessary to check that the abnormality seen on MRI correlates with the part of the brain producing the seizures.

● **A test called the sodium amytal** test is sometimes also carried out. This involves injecting the anaesthetic agent, sodium amytal, into each side of the brain in turn; the injection is through a tube inserted into the main blood vessel in the groin and then passed up to the blood vessels supplying the brain.

Although this sounds quite unpleasant, it is a relatively painless and safe procedure. As a result of the injection, each half of the brain is put to sleep in turn for a few minutes. During this period, the patient's memory and ability to name various objects are then tested. Failure to complete the tests accurately means that the half of the brain put to sleep controls language and memory.

In most people language resides in the left half of the brain and memory resides in both halves, but in a small number of people this pattern is lost. It is important to know if this is the case, because the effects of brain surgery on speech, understanding and memory are vital factors in deciding whether surgery is indicated and what type of operation is possible.

● **Lastly, it is common for a psychiatric assessment** to be performed in order to confirm that there is no mental illness present that would prevent the patient from having brain surgery (for example, very severe depression or suicidal tendencies). If a mental condition is discovered, this needs to be treated before surgery can be performed.

PSYCHIATRIC ASSESSMENT
Many patients will be required to visit a psychiatrist before surgery, in order to rule out any underlying mental illness.

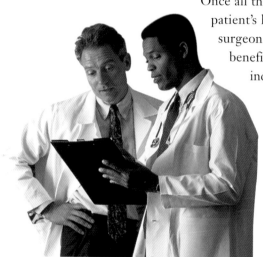

Once all this information is available, the patient's hospital doctors and the brain surgeon meet to discuss the risks and benefits of epilepsy surgery for each individual patient.

Once this has been decided, the risks and likely benefits are put to the patient, who then has to make a decision.

THE OUTCOME

The outcome for epilepsy surgery depends largely upon the type of operation, the part of the brain involved and the underlying cause of the epilepsy.

REACHING A CONCLUSION
Once all the tests have been completed, the risks and benefits of surgery for the patient are discussed by the doctor and surgeon.

In patients who have an identifiable defect in the temporal lobe of the brain (which is the most common situation), about 70 per cent of them will become seizure free after surgery, and another 20 per cent will have some improvement. This does, however, still leave one in 10 patients who has no improvement or who may even be worse. Nevertheless, with improved imaging and surgical techniques, the outcome of epilepsy surgery continues to improve.

KEY POINTS

- The aim of long-term treatment of epilepsy is to stop seizures.
- An antiepileptic drug is chosen to suit the patient.
- Side-effects of drugs can be dose-related, occur in only some individuals or occur only in the long term.
- Some patients with epilepsy benefit from brain surgery.

Drugs used in the treatment of epilepsy

Most people who experience epileptic seizures find that their symptoms can be controlled with anticonvulsant drug therapy. Some drugs have been around for many years, but others are much more recent.

ESTABLISHED DRUGS

Some of the most commonly used antiepileptic drugs have been in use since the early part of this century.

CARBAMAZEPINE

This drug has been around since the 1950s, and has been found to be both safe and effective in partial epilepsy and tonic-clonic seizures. It can, however, worsen absences and myoclonic jerks. Occasionally a rash or abnormalities of blood counts can occur that may mean that the drug has to be stopped. Too high a dose can lead to double vision, nausea, headache and drowsiness. Carbamazepine is also available as a slow-release preparation (once swallowed, the drug is only slowly released from the tablet), which can be taken less frequently and has fewer side-effects.

DRUG THERAPY
Most people find that their seizures can be controlled by taking either one of the more established drugs, or one of the new types of medication.

CLONAZEPAM

The drug Clonazepam is one of a group of drugs called benzodiazepines (others will be mentioned later), which are better known for their use in anxiety and as sleeping tablets. This drug is effective in absence seizures and other forms of epilepsy. However, in some patients the drug ceases to be effective after a period of time (usually about three months); this phenomenon is called tolerance. Like all benzodiazepines, drowsiness and behavioural changes (especially aggression in children) are the main side-effects.

ETHOSUXIMIDE

This drug is only useful in absence epilepsy. Some patients develop a rash, and side-effects can include stomach ache, tiredness, headache and dizziness.

PHENOBARBITONE

Phenobarbitone is one of the oldest of the established antiepileptic drugs, having been used since 1912. It is cheap and effective in most types of epilepsy, but in recent years it has grown out of favour due to its side-effects. Originally phenobarbitone was used as a sleeping pill; it is thus not surprising that some people become drowsy, although this drowsiness is slight and usually improves with time. Paradoxically, it can have the opposite effect in children, and make them hyperactive and aggressive. In a few, phenobarbitone can cause a rash and blistering. Too high a dose leads to drowsiness, impotence, depression and poor memory. With long-term use, phenobarbitone can coarsen facial features and decrease the body's stores of certain vitamins (folic acid and vitamin D).

PHENYTOIN

This drug has been in common usage since 1938. It was initially seen as a breakthrough because it was as effective as phenobarbitone but caused less drowsiness. Phenytoin is effective in partial seizures and tonic-clonic seizures. Some patients get a rash, in which case it should be stopped. Too high a dose can lead to dizziness, increased seizures, drowsiness, unsteadiness and double vision. Long-term use can lead to swelling of the gums, coarsening of facial features, acne, facial hair and a decrease in the body's stores of certain vitamins (folic acid and vitamin D). Because of these long-term side-effects, young people are not keen to use phenytoin and often a different antiepileptic drug is preferred.

WEIGHT GAIN
Some patients find that they put on weight when taking medication such as gabapentin or valproate.

PRIMIDONE

This drug is broken down in the body to phenobarbitone, and thus it has the same side-effects and uses as phenobarbitone.

VALPROATE

In France, in the 1960s, this drug was discovered to be useful in epilepsy purely by chance. It is now the drug of choice for light-sensitive epilepsy, myoclonic seizures and absences. It is, however, effective in all types of epilepsy. It needs to be used cautiously in children under the age of three years, when it very occasionally causes severe liver damage. Some people can get a drop in the number of platelets in the blood (these are necessary for blood clotting).

The most common side-effects, however, are stomach upset, hair loss, tremor, swelling of the ankles, weight gain and drowsiness (especially if given with phenobarbitone). Valproate is available as a slow release preparation.

NEWER DRUGS

When new antiepileptic drugs are first developed, they are tried on patients with uncontrolled epilepsy (usually partial epilepsy) as an add-on therapy to existing antiepileptic drug courses. If they prove to be successful, then initially they are licensed just for this purpose. Some new antiepileptic drugs are, however, effective in types of epilepsy that fall outside the scope of the licence. Doctors are permitted to prescribe drugs for such conditions, but they will usually discuss this with the patient first.

GABAPENTIN

At present, gabapentin is only licensed to be used in partial epilepsy in combination with other antiepileptic drugs. It has few side-effects, but at higher doses can cause dizziness, tremor and drowsiness; the frequency of seizures can also increase in some patients. The drug can also result in weight gain.

LAMOTRIGINE

This drug originally had the same restricted licence as gabapentin, but can now be used in a variety of different seizures and as monotherapy. It is potentially useful in most types of epilepsy. In a few patients, it causes a rash, and this seems to be more likely to occur if a patient is started at too high a dose. Too high a dose can cause drowsiness, double vision and dizziness.

Antiepileptic Drugs and Their Year of Introduction in the UK

Some of the drugs used in the treatment of epileptic seizures have been around since the turn of the century; others are fairly new.

DRUG (TRADE NAME)	YEAR OF INTRODUCTION
Phenobarbitone (Gardenal)	1912
Phenytoin (Epanutin)	1938
Primidone (Mysoline)	1952
Ethosuximide (Zarontin)	1960
Carbamazepine (Tegretol)	1963
Diazepam (Valium)	1973
Clonazepam (Rivotril)	1974
Valproate (Epilim)	1974
Clobazam (Frisium)	1982
Vigabatrin (Sabril)	1989
Slow-release carbamazepine (Tegretol Retard)	1989
Lamotrigine (Lamictal)	1991
Gabapentin (Neurontin)	1993
Slow-release valproate (Epilim Chrono)	1993
Topiramate (Topamax)	1995
Tiagabine (Gabatril)	1998
Fosphenytoin	1998

TOPIRAMATE

This is a recent antiepileptic drug that can be used as add-on treatment for a variety of seizure types. Its side-effects usually occur on starting treatment and include tiredness, stomach upset, unsteadiness and, rarely, kidney stones. Patients can also experience weight loss.

TIAGABINE

This is the most recent antiepileptic drug to gain a licence in the UK as add-on treatment for use in partial epilepsy. The drug's main side-effects are dizziness, tremor, tiredness, depression and, occasionally, diarrhoea.

VIGABATRIN

This drug is only licensed for partial epilepsy in combination with other antiepileptic drugs. However, it may also have some use in other forms of epilepsy in children. About one in 20 people get depression as a side- effect of the drug, and occasionally confusion or psychotic symptoms can occur.

Other side-effects such as drowsiness and dizziness are usually mild. Some patients also put on weight while taking vigabatrin.

There have been recent concerns of the effects of vigabatrin on vision, such that long-term vigabatrin use can result, in some patients, in tunnel vision. This has meant that doctors have not been so keen to start vigabatrin, and people on vigabatrin need their vision closely monitored.

OTHER DRUGS

Drugs that have been developed primarily for other conditions (for example diuretic drugs or drugs to treat anxiety and depression) have in some instances proved valuable in the treatment of epileptic seizures.

ACETAZOLAMIDE

This drug is a diuretic (a drug that makes you pass more urine), and it is mainly used to treat glaucoma (an eye condition). It is, however, occasionally used as additional medication for patients with epilepsy and, in some, it can be very effective.

The main problem is that after a few months, tolerance develops (i.e., the drug loses its ability to work effectively) in some patients; it can also cause a rash. The other main side effects are excessive thirst, tingling in the hands and feet, tiredness and loss of appetite.

CLOBAZAM

This is a benzodiazepine (see Clonazepam, p.53). It may be very effective in most types of epilepsy as an additional medication, but again tolerance develops in some patients after a few months. It is occasionally given intermittently (that is, for three or four days at a time) in those whose seizures occur in small groups (clusters), or at set times (for example, at the time of menstruation) or on days when it is particularly important to avoid a seizure.

DIAZEPAM

This drug is also a benzodiazepine and it is not usually used as regular medication, but as a one-off in order to stop a long seizure. For this purpose it can be given by mouth or by suppository by carers or family. In hospital, it can be given by intravenous infusion (i.e., directly into a vein) to stop prolonged seizures.

VITAMINS AND DIET

There is little evidence that either of these help seizures. Vitamin supplements may, however, be necessary for those on long-term antiepileptic drug treatment, because some antiepileptic drugs (see above) can interfere with the body's vitamin stores. Supplementary folic acid is also recommended for those who wish to get pregnant.

There is a high fat, low carbohydrate diet called a ketogenic diet, which may help seizure control in some children with severe epilepsy and mental handicap. Unfortunately this diet is unpleasant and difficult to maintain, so it is rarely used.

DRUGS FOR THE FUTURE

There are at present many studies taking place throughout the world of potential antiepileptic drugs (at the time of writing, at least ten new compounds look quite promising). This is encouraging for the future of antiepileptic drug treatment. However, no drug so far has proved to be a cure-all, and one of the unanswered questions for epilepsy research is why only some patients respond to only some drugs. Nevertheless, each new drug enables a greater number of patients to have a significant improvement in their epilepsy. It is hoped that, with a greater armoury of drugs, fewer people will have uncontrolled seizures.

The newer drugs may have fewer side-effects than the older drugs, but it is important to realise that long-term side-effects of new drugs may be unrecognised in contrast to those of older drugs, some of which have been around for over 50 years.

KEY POINTS

- Antiepileptic medication will help control seizures in most people.
- Some of the drugs used have been around since the turn of the century.

Special situations

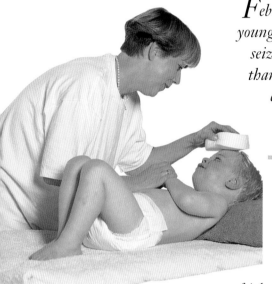

Febrile convulsions (experienced by young children) and status epilepticus seizure (a seizure that lasts more than 30 minutes) have particular characteristics that require a special explanation.

▬ FEBRILE CONVULSIONS ▬

This term is usually reserved for convulsions that occur in young children (three months to five years) only at the time of fever ('febrile'). Febrile convulsions are important because they are common and often frightening. It should not, however, be referred to as epilepsy, because the condition almost always resolves as the child grows older.

CONVULSIONS IN CHILDREN
A high fever may cause a febrile convulsion in a young child so it is important to try to reduce a high temperature by, for example, sponging with lukewarm water.

It is sometimes necessary to exclude brain infections such as meningitis as a cause, and occasionally a 'lumbar puncture' (in which a needle is inserted into the spine of a child in order to withdraw some of the fluid that surrounds the brain) is needed to make sure that there is no brain infection. In most cases there is no meningitis or other serious cause.

Indeed, over three per cent of children between the ages of three months and five years will have at least one seizure associated with fever without underlying brain disease. It is more common in those with a relative who has had similar seizures or who has epilepsy. One-third of children who have a febrile convulsion have subsequent febrile convulsions, but a very small number (less than five per cent) go on to develop true epilepsy.

If a child has had a convulsion with fever, then in future febrile episodes the child's temperature should be kept down with paracetamol and cold sponging. In very susceptible children, diazepam suppositories can be given at the time of a fever to prevent another convulsion, and, very rarely, a child may need regular antiepileptic medication, usually with valproate or phenobarbitone.

How a Lumbar Puncture is Performed

A needle is inserted into the base of the spine to obtain a sample of cerebrospinal fluid. Examination of the cerebrospinal fluid can help in the diagnosis of such diseases as meningitis.

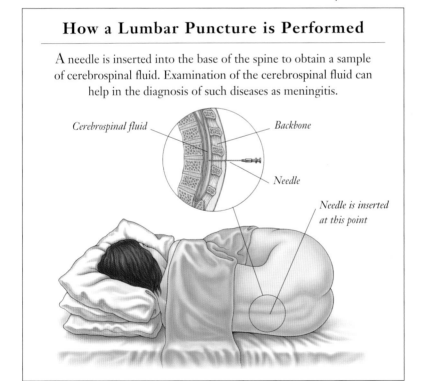

Cerebrospinal fluid

Backbone

Needle

Needle is inserted at this point

STATUS EPILEPTICUS

Most seizures only last a few minutes. Some, however, can go on for longer – sometimes hours or even days. This is referred to as status epilepticus, which is defined as a seizure or a series of seizures lasting more than 30 minutes in which the patient does not regain consciousness. This can apply to all seizure types; tonic-clonic status epilepticus (usually called convulsive status epilepticus) is of most important because it is a medical emergency.

As many as 10 per cent of patients with convulsive status epilepticus die (usually not as a result of the epilepsy itself, but of the serious underlying cause of the status epilepticus, e.g. meningitis, stroke or malignant brain tumours). About half the patients with status epilepticus have had chronic epilepsy; in these cases, sudden withdrawal of the antiepileptic drug is one of the most common identifiable causes. About half the patients have convulsive status epilepticus as their first seizure. When it occurs, urgent hospitalisation and emergency, intravenous, antiepileptic drug therapy are required.

Many patients have increasing numbers of seizures throughout the day leading up to the convulsive status epilepticus, and in some (certainly those in whom status epilepticus occurs regularly) diazepam, given by mouth or suppository, will prevent the occurrence of the status epilepticus. Such a contingency plan needs to be made between the doctor and the carers or the family of the patient concerned.

The other, non-convulsive types of status epilepticus are not as serious. Often the patient will just have a prolonged typical seizure or series of seizures, leading to confusion that can go on for days. Non-convulsive status epilepticus usually responds well to medication given by mouth (often diazepam).

PREGNANCY AND EPILEPSY

Careful monitoring of drug levels and frequency of seizures is necessary during pregnancy to ensure the health and well-being of both mother and baby.

CONCEPTION

Patients with epilepsy have lower birth rates. This is primarily due to social pressures, although epilepsy and its treatment can occasionally affect fertility. Furthermore, some antiepileptic drugs may have the effect of decreasing sexual drive.

The effectiveness of the contraceptive pill can be reduced by antiepileptic drugs, and higher doses of the pill may be necessary in order to provide adequate contraception. Bleeding between menstrual periods is a useful sign that the oral contraceptive is not working.

PREGNANCY

During pregnancy, about 30 per cent of patients experience an increase in seizures, 20 per cent experience a decrease in seizures and 50 per cent experience no change. The way the body deals with antiepileptic drugs is different during pregnancy, and regular monitoring of drug levels and seizures is often required. Quite often the dose of antiepileptic drugs has to be changed at some point during pregnancy. It is not uncommon for the mother to decide to reduce her medication during pregnancy because of a concern about the effects of the antiepileptic drugs on the developing child. Major, convulsive seizures can, however, damage the developing child or result in miscarriage, and thus the importance of good compliance cannot be over-emphasised.

The risks of antiepileptic drugs to the development of the baby in the womb are small. The risk is higher in infants born to mothers on polytherapy and on high doses of antiepileptic drugs. The overall frequency of abnormalities of the baby at birth is about two per cent for the general population, six per cent for babies born to mothers on one antiepileptic drug (i.e. still quite small) and up to 20 per cent for babies born to mothers on three different antiepileptic drugs (i.e. quite high). Thus, before getting pregnant, it is important for the doctor to get the patient on to the minimum amount of medication for adequate control of the epilepsy.

The most common significant abnormality in infants born to mothers with epilepsy is cleft lip/palate, which accounts for about one-third of the abnormalities seen. Spina bifida, the more serious side-effect of drug treatment, is most common when the mother is taking valproate (1–2 per cent of births) or carbamazepine (0.5–1 per cent of births). Patients on these drugs can have ultrasound and blood tests during pregnancy to detect spina bifida early enough for the pregnancy to be safely terminated, if the parents wish. All women on antiepileptic drugs should be given folic acid tablets (this is a naturally occurring vitamin) before conception and throughout the first three months of pregnancy, because this reduces the risk of miscarriage and fetal malformation, especially spina bifida (there is an argument for all women to take folic acid during these periods regardless of whether they have epilepsy or not). In the last month of pregnancy vitamin K supplements

CLOSE MONITORING
Medication must be carefully monitored during pregnancy to ensure that no harm comes to either the mother or the unborn baby.

should be given to the mother, and the newborn child should also receive vitamin K because antiepileptic drugs decrease the amount of this vitamin in the body. If the newborn child does not have enough vitamin K, then the blood may not clot properly, and there may be problems with bleeding and brain haemorrhage.

BREAST-FEEDING
Women with epilepsy on antiepileptic drugs usually can safely breast-feed, because with most antiepileptic drugs very little is passed out into breast milk. The exceptions are high doses of ethosuximide or phenobarbitone, which are excreted in breast milk in significant quantities; phenobarbitone excreted into breast milk can make the baby drowsy.

KEY POINTS

- Convulsions that occur in young children only at the time of a fever do not usually lead to epilepsy.
- Seizures that last for hours or days are known as status epilepticus. Convulsive status epilepticus is a medical emergency.
- During pregnancy, the risks of antiepileptic drugs to the baby are small, and certainly smaller than the risks of the mother having uncontrolled convulsions.
- It is generally safe for women to breast-feed while taking anticonvulsants.

The social implications

Although we have spent a large part of this book dealing with the medical aspects of epilepsy, it is important to realise that there are many social implications of epilepsy, for instance in regard to driving, schooling, employment and relationships.

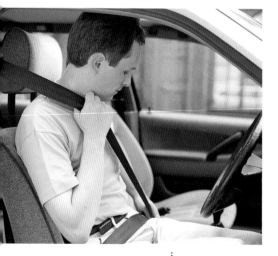

Unfortunately, society still places extra pressures on those who have epilepsy, though sometimes with some justification, as in the case of driving.

DRIVING

Seizures while driving are still one of the most common preventable causes of road traffic accidents. The rules laid down about driving are very straightforward, and there is little excuse not to follow them. It is the obligation and responsibility of every person who has any condition that may impede his or her driving (this includes all people with epilepsy) to inform the Driver and Vehicle Licensing Authority (DVLA). Anyone who fails to inform the DVLA, and continues to drive, is committing a criminal offence. Furthermore, failing to inform the DVLA may invalidate the driving insurance. This applies to all people with seizures, and for this purpose even the smallest epileptic event (for example, an aura or a myoclonic jerk) is counted as a seizure.

Once the DVLA has been informed, the patient should stop driving and can reapply for a licence only when one of the criteria in the box has been fulfilled.

DVLA Criteria for Driving

Reapplication for a driving licence can only be considered by the DVLA when either of the criteria below is fulfilled:

- No epileptic attacks (this also includes aura, etc.) have occurred during the previous year.
- Epileptic attacks have occurred in the last three years only during periods of sleep.

Following a single epileptic seizure, or if there is loss of consciousness of no known cause, patients can also be barred from driving for one year. When reapplying for a licence, it is necessary for the patient to fill in a detailed form about the attacks, and the DVLA can also seek information from the patient's GP and hospital specialist. If any person is unhappy with the DVLA's decision, it is possible to appeal through a Magistrates' court.

If a patient has been seizure free, and has thus regained his driving licence, but wishes to come off medication, it is advised that the patient should not drive during the changes in medication and for six months after the withdrawal, although this is not legally binding. Unfortunately, a seizure that occurs while coming off medication will result in loss of the licence.

The rules for heavy goods vehicle (HGV) and passenger carrying vehicle (PCV) licences are much stricter, and it is not possible to hold these licences if a person has a continuing liability to epileptic seizures.

This is interpreted as meaning no epileptic seizure or antiepileptic medication for the previous 10 years and no medical evidence of a continuing risk of seizures (e.g. three per second spike and wave on the EEG or a brain abnormality on a brain scan).

EMPLOYMENT

There are a few occupations that are barred by statutory provision for people with epilepsy. These are aircraft

EXCLUDED PROFESSIONS
Unfortunately, people with epilepsy cannot become airline pilots, as a seizure while working would obviously put others in considerable danger.

pilot, ambulance driver, taxi driver, train driver, merchant seaman and anyone working in the armed services, fire brigade or police.

There are also certain jobs that involve substantial risks if a seizure should occur, and therefore cannot be recommended (e.g. scaffolder), and commonsense should apply when considering such jobs. Furthermore, there are jobs in which epilepsy is not explicitly mentioned but may be considered a bar (e.g. midwifery).

Patients are under an obligation to tell employers if they have epilepsy, if this could affect their ability to do the job, or affect their safety at work. Failure to disclose epilepsy in such circumstances can be used as grounds for dismissal.

If a seizure is likely to occur at work, it is, in our view, probably better to tell an employer rather than keep the epilepsy secret. If an employer is aware of a person's epilepsy and takes it into consideration, then the work insurance will cover that person, regardless of his condition. It is important to tell a workmate if a seizure is likely to occur at work, and to explain what to do if a seizure should occur.

When initially applying for a job, unless the epilepsy is likely to have a severe effect on the ability to do the job, there is no obligation to inform possible employers unless specifically asked. If asked on forms, it is important not to over-emphasise the epilepsy and in some cases it may be advisable to leave that section blank or to write that it will be discussed at interview. The best moments for mentioning epilepsy are just before accepting the job offer or at final interview, but again it is important to try to place it in a favourable light. Often a letter from the GP or hospital doctor will help. The prejudice perceived by people with epilepsy when applying for jobs is probably often greater than the actual prejudice. Some people blame their failure to get work on their epilepsy when, in fact, the problem lies more in the person's attitude; it is essential at interview to appear confident, and appropriate for the job, rather than dwell too much on the negative aspects of epilepsy.

ASSESSING THE RISKS

One of the most important features of epilepsy is that it is an intermittent condition. If someone has a seizure once a week (this would be considered as poorly controlled epilepsy), it still leaves 313 days in a year when the person is seizure-free. It is thus important that a person does not let the epilepsy take over and dictate his or her life. Overprotection, excessive restrictions and under-achievement are far too common secondary handicaps of epilepsy, which can be avoided. The main dangers from epilepsy come from its unpredictability, and certain precautions need to be taken.

ACTIVITES TO AVOID
High-risk sports, such as scuba-diving, should be avoided as seizures cannot be predicted.

It would be prudent to avoid certain high-risk situations such as mountain climbing, scuba diving and hang-gliding (although well-organised mountain climbs are possible).

In most other circumstances, the social and psychological damage done by restricting a person's life probably outstrip the risks. Swimming is perfectly possible, but preferably with someone who knows about the epilepsy and knows what to do should a seizure occur, and the pool attendant should be informed. Cycling and horse riding are perfectly possible, but again attention should be paid to the possible risks; both these pursuits need to be done either with someone who knows about the epilepsy or in an organised group, and a helmet is mandatory.

At home, most activities carry only a small risk. There are, however, certain actions that can be taken to minimise these risks. Showers should be preferred to baths and, if a bath is taken, it should be shallow and someone should be informed. Additionally, the bathroom door should remain unlocked. A microwave is preferable to a cooker, and pans of hot oil should be avoided. Guards for open fires, radiators and cookers are advisable. Lastly, there are alarms that are available for people with epilepsy, which are triggered if, for example, the person falls; these are useful for people with frequent seizures who are living alone.

Frequent falls in someone with poorly controlled epilepsy can cause head and facial injuries. If these falls continue for long enough, then a certain amount of brain damage and facial scarring can occur. In these people (very much the minority of people who have epilepsy), a protective helmet is advisable.

SCHOOLING AND PARENTING

It is wrong to generalise about a child with epilepsy. Epilepsy, as we hope is now apparent, describes many different conditions, has many different underlying causes and occurs in many different people. It is inexcusable to label a person with epilepsy as an epileptic child or an epileptic adult, and thus to suggest a stereotype. Despite this, there are some important points about schooling that need to be made.

Most children with epilepsy attend normal schools, and only the minority, who have epilepsy and learning difficulties or very severe epilepsy, need to attend special schools (advice about these is available from a number of organizations – see Useful addresses, pp.80–81). Despite attending mainstream education, many children with epilepsy underachieve at school for a variety of reasons. Epilepsy itself and antiepileptic drugs can impair a child's ability to learn. However, with modern drug management, there is less impairment of memory and greater control of seizures. A child with absence epilepsy can have many seizures that are unrecognised by both child and teacher, but which can present as lapses of concentration and poor class performance. Seizures at night can also affect performance during the day.

More importantly, many children with epilepsy are almost expected by some to perform poorly, and this expectation by parents and teachers soon becomes self-fulfilling. Poor school attendance, low self-esteem and anxieties about school are all likely to be major factors.

GOING TO SCHOOL
Most children with epilepsy are able to attend mainstream schools.

71

There has to be good communication between school, parents, child and doctor. It is important that the school knows about the epilepsy, that teachers know what to do about seizures and that they understand a child's condition. Education packages for schools are available from a number of charitable organizations (see Useful addresses, pp.80–81).

In addition, it is important that neither teachers nor parents restrict the activities of a child unnecessarily (see Assessing the risks, pp.69–70). The child should be encouraged to think positively and to take part in school activities. Teachers should be aware of possible teasing and bullying. If it is likely that a child will have a seizure at school, then often it is worth educating the class about seizures and epilepsy. It is important that the child does not feel, or indeed become, isolated because of his or her seizures.

Over-protection by families, even in well-controlled epilepsy, let alone in poorly controlled epilepsy, is very common and is counter-productive. This over-protection, which often persists into adulthood, can result in social isolation, poor social graces, dependency, childishness, underachievement and low self-esteem. Striking a balance is understandably difficult, but it is important that this issue is not ignored. Parents should not be afraid to discuss their child's epilepsy with doctors, counsellors or others in order to have a better understanding not only of their child's epilepsy, but also of the restrictions that this will impose upon their child's life. In our experience, parents tend to verge much too much on the side of over-vigilance and over-anxiety, and therefore the potential for both psychological and social damage is great.

RELATIONSHIPS

In broad terms, people with epilepsy have fewer relationships and are often more isolated than is normal. Prejudice among the general public is often blamed, but the actual causes of this are more complex. Some patients believe that there is a greater prejudice than actually exists. This, in combination with parental over-protection, can lead to a fear of relationships, and this anxiety often makes forming relationships more difficult. This results in a certain amount of social isolation that serves to fuel the original anxieties. We often find that these worries remain even when patients become seizure-free. Many people with epilepsy thus need to be encouraged to think positively about themselves and their condition, and to face their anxieties. Occasionally help is needed, and advice about this is available from a number of sources (see pp.80–81). It is important not to let epilepsy dominate one's life inappropriately, as such a preoccupation can be very self-destructive.

Once in a relationship, if the epilepsy is still active it is important that the partner is aware of this. There is no evidence to suggest that knowledge of a person's epilepsy is a major cause in the break up of relationships. Although this may sound an obvious recommendation, we are certainly aware of one person whose wife discovered about his epilepsy for the first time during a honeymoon night. How and when to tell a partner can be difficult, but again the positive aspects of the condition should be emphasised – usually epilepsy is easily controlled, it is not inherited, it does not lead to mental illness, etc. It is also perfectly

A TRUE PARTNERSHIP
There is no reason why someone with epilepsy should not enjoy a loving, fulfilling relationship. It may be difficult to tell a partner about your epilepsy but it important to emphasis the positive aspects of the disease.

possible to have a family (see p.63), and for people with active epilepsy to look after and bring up children. There is a danger of over-dependency in some relationships, and of treating the affected partner as a child; both of these should be avoided.

PSYCHIATRIC DISEASE

The connection between psychiatric disease and seizures is complex. In the past, epilepsy was viewed as a form of psychiatric disease, but now it is considered a physical brain disease.

Psychiatric disease is, however, not uncommon in people with epilepsy. A person with epilepsy faces many social pressures, and is more likely to be unemployed and single. It is therefore not surprising that anxiety and depression are common in those with epilepsy, especially those with a long history of poorly controlled seizures. However, both seizures and antiepileptic drugs can compound this depression through their effects on the brain, and can occasionally themselves produce a very severe depression that may require hospitalization and drug treatment.

Rarely, patients with temporal lobe epilepsy have episodes of paranoia and schizophrenic-like illnesses. These episodes are usually short-lived occurring around the time of a seizure, just after a seizure or between seizures. In a few individuals these episodes may persist, and may require long-term drug treatment. The exact association between temporal lobe epilepsy and psychosis is unclear, because both increases in seizure frequency (flurries of seizures) and decreases in seizure frequency can in some cases result in psychotic episodes in some unfortunate people.

Some psychiatric diseases and epilepsy have a common cause, for instance severe brain damage at birth may lead to seizures, personality problems and psychiatric disease. In these cases, it is not the epilepsy that causes the psychiatric problems but an underlying cause that results in both conditions.

KEY POINTS

- All people who have a driving licence need to inform the DVLA if they develop epileptic seizures.
- It is best to inform your employer if you have epilepsy.
- High-risk situations such as strenuous or dangerous sports should be avoided; most sports can be enjoyed under some supervision.
- Parents of children with epilepsy should not be over-protective because this can result in their child's social isolation.
- Forming relationships can occasionally be difficult for people with epilepsy, but people with epilepsy must be careful not to let the condition 'control' their lives.

Overall outlook

With the appropriate care and treatment, most people with epilepsy can look forward to leading a normal and fulfilling life, with a normal life expectancy.

THE LIKELY OUTCOME

The outlook or prognosis of a condition is the 'forecast' for that condition; it tells us what is going to happen in the future. As was described in the introduction, epilepsy resolves in most people, and can thus be said to have a good prognosis. About 80 per cent of people on antiepileptic medication become seizure-free, and there thus has to be the decision about when to stop the medication. It is usual to wait for a patient to be seizure free for roughly two years before

A POSITIVE OUTLOOK
Young people are more likely to remain seizure-free than adults when medication is stopped.

stopping medication. There are a number of factors that determine the chances of success or failure in withdrawing drugs, including the underlying cause of the epilepsy. Overall, however, about 60 per cent of patients who have been seizure-free for two years successfully come off drugs.

The chances of coming off medication are better in the young, and in those taking only one antiepileptic drug.

Some people do not wish to risk coming off their drugs, because the social consequences of having a seizure may be too great (loss of driving licence, etc.).

These social consequences tend to be greater in adults than in children. Indeed, because of the better chances of withdrawing medication, the lesser consequences of having a seizure and the effects of medication on schooling, seizure-free children are often the group that benefit most from coming off their antiepileptic drugs.

One of the questions that has been the subject of debate for many years is whether antiepileptic drugs themselves help cure the condition as well as stopping seizures. The answer to this question is unknown. Recently, however, studies have demonstrated that even late antiepileptic drug treatment probably carries the same good prognosis as early drug treatment.

MENTAL AND PHYSICAL HEALTH

There is often concern that epilepsy and seizures commonly lead to mental and physical deterioration. This is not so. In most cases, seizures either stop or are well-controlled by antiepileptic drugs, and these people usually lead normal lives. Unfortunately, there are a few who have uncontrolled seizures, in whom mental and physical deterioration may occasionally be seen. In these cases, however, the deterioration is usually due to the underlying cause of the epilepsy or injuries that occur during the seizures rather than the seizures themselves.

The possible development of mental illness is often another concern, but, as has already been explained, mental illness directly attributable to seizures is rare, and seizures themselves rarely lead to the destruction of personality and mind.

77

DEATH AND EPILEPSY

Does epilepsy affect life expectancy? The answer is that poorly controlled, severe epilepsy most certainly does, and even people with well-controlled epilepsy may have a slightly shortened life expectancy. The reasons for this are not altogether certain, but in a number of cases the underlying cause of the epilepsy (e.g., a brain tumour) may obviously shorten life expectancy. In addition, people with epilepsy are at a higher risk of accidents, usually while having a seizure or as the result of the seizure. Sudden unexpected death, which is a sudden unwitnessed death in a previously healthy person for which no cause is found post mortem, is more common in epilepsy and may be as high as one in 400 people with epilepsy per year (probably even higher in people with severe epilepsy). The reasons for this are again unclear, but it may be the result of an unwitnessed seizure.

Having said this, most seizures do not result in death or brain damage. It is certain, however, that people with well-controlled epilepsy do better than those with poorly controlled epilepsy, and as treatment continues to improve, so the prognosis for epilepsy, the lives and even the life expectancy of those with epilepsy improve along with it.

KEY POINTS

- Epilepsy resolves in most people.
- People with epilepsy can reduce or prevent their seizures with drugs and can then lead normal lives.
- Seizures rarely cause brain damage or death.

Summary

In this book there are a number of important points that we would like to emphasise.

- Epilepsy is a common and treatable condition.
- A seizure results from an 'electrical storm' in the brain, and the form of a seizure depends on where it starts and how far it spreads.
- A number of conditions can be confused with seizures.
- There are a multitude of causes of seizures.
- Febrile convulsions rarely lead to epilepsy.
- Most people with epilepsy are well-controlled with drug treatment, which must be taken regularly.
- Doses of antiepileptic drugs are determined by the balance of seizure control against drug side-effects.
- Antiepileptic blood levels are merely a guide to drug doses.
- Epilepsy gets better and 'goes away' in many people.
- The prognosis probably relates to the underlying cause of the epilepsy.
- Brain surgery is successful in, and suitable for, a number of patients with drug-resistant epilepsy.
- Most prejudice against people with epilepsy is unjust, but often it is not as great as the person with epilepsy believes.
- Most people with epilepsy should lead normal lives, and should not be over-protected.
- Lastly, epileptic is an adjective that should be confined to the phrase 'epileptic seizure' and not be used to describe and stereotype people.

Useful addresses

ASSESSMENT CENTRES FOR EPILEPSY

In the UK there are a number of specialist assessment centres for epilepsy. Two have been designated for adults (The National Society for Epilepsy, and Bootham Park Hospital) and one for children (Park Hospital for Children). There are, however, other specialist epilepsy units, including National Hospital for Neurology and Neurosurgery, David Lewis Centre and King's College Hospital. In addition to these, there are specialist units in many regional neurological centres. These units specialise in the assessment of patients with epilepsy, especially those patients who are resistant to antiepileptic drug treatment.

David Lewis Organisation
Mill Lane
Warford
Alderley Edge
Mobberley
Cheshire SK9 7UD
Tel: (01565) 640000

King's College Hospital – Epilepsy Unit
Denmark Hill
London SE5 9ES
Tel: (0171) 346 5354

National Hospital for Neurology and Neurosurgery – Epilepsy Unit
Queen Square
London WC1N 3BG
Tel: (0171) 837 3611

The National Society for Epilepsy
Chalfont Centre for Epilepsy
Chalfont St. Peter
Buckinghamshire SL9 ORJ
Tel: (01494) 601300
Helpline: (01494) 601 400

Park Hospital for Children
Old Road
Headington
Oxford OX3 7LQ
Tel: (01865) 741717

Special Centre for Epilepsy
York District Hospital
Wigginton Road
York YO3 7HE
Tel: (01904) 454161

SPECIAL SCHOOLS FOR CHILDREN WITH EPILEPSY

Most children with epilepsy receive mainstream schooling. There are, however, children with severe epilepsy, learning difficulties or behavioural problems that preclude them from mainstream education.

These children are often eligible for residential schooling in a specialist centre where there is medical supervision. A list is given on the following page.

David Lewis Organisation
Mill Lane
Warford
Alderley Edge
Mobberley,
Cheshire SK9 7UD
Tel: (01565) 640000

St. Piers School
St. Piers Lane
Lingfield
Surrey RH7 6PW
Tel: (01342) 832243

St. Elizabeth's Home
South End
Bourne Lane
Much Hadham
Hertfordshire SG10 6EW
Tel: (0127) 984 3451

EPILEPSY ORGANISATIONS
There are a number of charitable organisations
(listed below) that are involved in providing
information about epilepsy, educating the
general public about epilepsy, organising
meetings and funding research. Some of these
organisations are able to provide videos and
information packages for schools. They also
run information services. The National Society
for Epilepsy is the main association in the UK,
and has a local community network.

National Society for Epilepsy
Chalfont Centre for Epilepsy
Chalfont St. Peter
Buckinghamshire SL9 ORJ
Tel:(01494) 601300

Also:
British Epilepsy Association
Anstey House
40 Hanover Square
Leeds LS3 1BE
Tel: (0113) 2439393

Croydon Epilepsy Society
Stanley Mews
71 Stanley Roa
Croydon CRO 3QF
Tel: (0181) 665 1255

Epilepsy Association of Scotland
National Headquarters
48 Govan Road
Glasgow G51 1JL
Tel: (0141) 427 4911

Irish Epilepsy Association
249 Crumlin Road
Dublin 12
Eire
Tel: (00 353) 1455 7500

Mersey Region Epilepsy Association
Glaxo Neurological Centre
Norton Street
Liverpool L3 8LR
Tel: (0151) 298 2666

Wales Epilepsy Association
15 Chester Street
St. Asaph
Denbighshire, LL17 ORE
Tel: (01745) 584444
Helpline: (0345) 413774

Glossary

Amytal test: an injection of sodium amytal (an anaesthetic) into the blood supply to each half of the brain in turn in order to determine the possible effects of epilepsy surgery on memory and language.

Aura: the warning that may occur before a major seizure, or it may occur in isolation; it is a simple partial seizure.

Compliance: the act of taking a drug as instructed.

Computed tomography (CT): a brain scan using X-rays and computer analysis to form detailed pictures of slices through the brain.

Dysplasia: the abnormal development of cells in the brain in this context.

Electroencephalography (EEG): the recording of brain waves (the electrical activity within the brain).

Epileptic seizures: also known as fits, they are the result of an electrical storm in the brain. They are divided into partial seizures (simple partial, complex partial and secondary generalized), which begin in one part of the brain but can spread to other parts, and generalized seizures (tonic-clonic, clonic, tonic, absences and myoclonus), which begin in both halves of the brain at once.

Febrile convulsions: fits that occur in children at the time of fever; they rarely lead to epilepsy.

Hemispheres: the two halves of the brain. In most of us the left half is 'dominant' and controls language.

Hippocampus: a part of the temporal lobe (see **Lobes**), which is involved in the formation of memories and which, if damaged, commonly causes epilepsy.

Hyperventilation: overbreathing, which can occasionally be confused with an epileptic seizure.

Idiosyncratic side-effects: side-effects that occur in only certain people – the most common side- effect with antiepileptic drugs is rash.

Lobes: different parts of the brain determined by position, and each lobe has a particular set of functions; the frontal lobe is at the front and deals with movement, the parietal lobe is in the middle and deals with sensation, the occipital lobe is at the back and deals with sight and the temporal lobe is at the side and deals with memory formation.

Magnetic resonance imaging (MRI): the use of a strong magnetic field and radio waves to cause the vibration of atoms that give off energy, which is then turned into a very detailed picture of the brain by computer analysis. MRI is much better than CT at detecting brain abnormalities that cause epilepsy.

Monotherapy: the taking of one drug.

Pharmacoresistant epilepsy: also known as refractory or drug-resistant epilepsy and is epilepsy that is resistant to antiepileptic drug therapy (this applies only to the minority of people with epilepsy).

Photosensitivity: present in about one in 20 people with epilepsy, and is the propensity to have a seizure brought on by flashing lights.

Polytherapy: the taking of two or more drugs.

Prognosis: the 'forecast' for a condition.

Pseudoseizures: seizures that are not epileptic but which are like an emotional outburst and are usually due to deep-rooted psychological problems. They do not respond to antiepileptic drug treatment, and can be difficult to tell apart from epileptic seizures.

Status epilepticus: a seizure, or series of seizures, without consciousness being regained that continues for over 30 minutes. If the seizure is a convulsion (convulsive status epilepticus), then this is a medical emergency, and the patient should be taken to hospital.

Syncope: a faint.

Video telemetry: the simultaneous recording of EEG with video, and is used in difficult to diagnose patients and for assessment before epilepsy surgery.

Index